THE WISDOM WAY
BOOK 1

(Part I of
Harmonic Power Series)

A REALLY INTERESTING BOOK
WHICH CAN HELP YOU LIVE
LONGER AND BETTER.

Your 141 day guide
to looking younger
and feeling better.

By following these simple guidelines and pointers to a more healthy and enjoyable life, you will begin to undo many of the stresses imposed by your lifestyle.

As you progress through the next 141 days, you will begin to feel more energised and look progressively younger.

Some of the tips and suggestions may, at first, seem obvious and some even pointless, but please persevere as they are all important and each forms a part of the whole new philosophy which delivers amazing benefits.

This 141 day programme is designed to change ingrained bad habits and 'convenient' lifestyles – using new information to inform your beliefs.

It will help you change for the better.

CONTENTS

CONTENTS (cont.)

CONTENTS (cont.)

CONTENTS (cont.)

CONTENTS (cont.)

CONTENTS (cont.)

CONTENTS (cont.)

1. SALT

Replace your table salt and your cooking salt with sea salt (or natural rock salt).

Sea salt contains a wide range of minerals and trace elements that benefit your body in a wide variety of ways. For example, there's one they collect in France (off the Atlantic cost) that is renowned for increasing sexual potency!

Human blood is said to have the same mineral and saline content as did sea water in the Carboniferous era. Sea salt and other natural products that help maintain or mimic this are of benefit to our health in an increasingly artificial world. YOU NEED THE IODINE!

For an analysis of sea salt see the article: "Salt: From white gold to white poison" *Caduceus*, No. 65 Winter 2004, p 29 to 35.

2.   SUGAR

White sugar is, as they say, "fine white and deadly", whereas brown sugar is a naturally occurring resource which, in <u>small</u> quantities, is good for you.

Your body must balance sweet with sour in order to maintain a healthy pH balance and combat infection. The excess of sugar in every aspect of our diet means that your blood stream is too acidic. This allows yeast and malignant bacteria to grow in your body's far-flung systems, building up or storing up problems for the future. Remove sugar from your diet and you will become much more healthy and have a lot more energy. You will also notice an increase in mental acuity.

3.   BREAD

Replace white bread in your diet with brown wholemeal bread. White bread is "refined" which means that they take out the bran, wheat germ etc and bleach the residual flour white to make it more attractive.

You need the whole grain to get the full benefit otherwise you are paying for a not very nutritious "mush".

Different types of flours (e.g. wheat, rye, spelt etc) have varying gluten content. If you are gluten sensitive use a low gluten flour / bread.

For further information on gluten sensitivity and intolerance, "*Wheat Belly*" by Dr. William Davis is very useful.

4.   WASH FRUIT

Always thoroughly wash fruit in a strong mixture of vinegar and warm water. This helps remove pesticide residues which can build up in your body and damage your health.

Fruit reaching your table has been sprayed as many as 19 times with toxins designed to kill insects, small mammals, frogs, birds and fungi. Any of these toxins will kill you if taken in a spoonful and whilst the residue on fruit is small it builds up over a period to a toxic load that your liver has trouble in dealing with.

Washing in warm water and acetic acid (that is vinegar) help to reduce this. They also warm up the fruit which has usually been kept in cold store, so helping stimulate enzymic activity and ripening.

5. MILK

Replace cow's milk in your diet with goat's milk or sheep's milk. Apart from being stuffed full of hormones and antibiotics put into the dairy feed to make them grow and try to keep them healthy in hellish conditions, cow's milk is not good for humans. The molecules are too big for easy digestion and it can cause congestion in your system.

It causes mucus to accumulate. Goat's milk is surprisingly nice once you try it and it is much better for you.

6.   FOOD INTAKE

Eat less food!

Most of us overeat out of habit and this puts a heavy, tiring load on the digestive system which is not designed to work at full capacity all the time.

If you cut down your food intake you will live longer! Luigi Cornaro, an Italian nobleman who lived 400 years ago in Padua, died in complete comfort aged 102. He wrote: "It is in everyone's power to eat and drink what is wholesome and avoid overfeeding. He that is wise enough to observe this will suffer little from other incapacities. The man who pursues a temperate life with all possible exactness will seldom, if ever, be seized with a disease." And if you simply reduce the size of your meals you will save money (and you won't feel hungry).

7. WALKING

Walk 3 miles a day. The veins in your legs are fitted with one-way valves so that when you walk the pressure of your weight on the veins on the underside of your feet, helps pump blood back up to your heart. This reduces the amount of work that your heart has to do. Also walking is very calming and it helps a number of the body's systems (particularly the stomach) to work better.

8.   RAW FOOD (see 75)

Eat some ripe raw vegetables every day. Be they a salad, a shredded carrot, some tomatoes, radishes, spring onions or artichokes etc.

Your body relies, to some extent, on the replacement of its digestive enzyme reservoir from the input of enzymes in raw food.

Cooking kills enzymes so you need to "top up" with raw food.

Reference – *"Food Enzymes"* The Missing Link to Radiant Health by Humbart Santillo, MHND. ISBN 0-934252-40-8. Hohm Press Box 2501 Prescott, Arizona 86302.

9. TRICKLE FEED

Human beings, like all the great apes, are "trickle feeders" in their "wild" state.

Instead of 3 square meals a day, get into the habit of eating a little and often.

This way you don't get hungry and your digestive system doesn't have to struggle with a heavy overload after big meals, but can function at its best.

You will lose weight this way and suffer less colds and minor ailments since your immune system, which is linked to your digestive system, will work better.

REMEMBER YOU ARE NOT THE BIN!

10. DEHYDRATION

Drink lots of fresh pure water, particularly when eating dry or preserved food. A healthy digestive system needs lots of water and relies for part of its intake on the water content of the food you eat. This, coupled with your saliva, your pancreatic and gastric juices, is vital to good digestive health which is the foundation of life. You need at least 3 litres a day. Most people get about half that and are dehydrated. Dehydration means dry lips, wrinkles, a sluggish system and a build up of toxins. Drink the water of life!

11. BITTERS

Because our modern diet is drenched with huge amounts of sugar, salt, emulsifiers and "e" numbers and so forth, we are all too sweet. We carry a heavy load of food additives and food conditioners which make our systems too acidic. Apart from reducing the pH of our blood, making it less able to transport sufficient oxygen to the extremities of our systems, this environment encourages parasites. Almost everybody who eats a modern western diet carries parasites (flukes, worms etc.) these probably won't kill you but they sap your strength and reduce your vitality.

I take 2 wormwood capsules and swallow them with a drink of water every morning. Otherwise you can use Swedish bitters each day or have a strong weekly dose of bitters to help get rid of worms and parasites and rebalance your system.

12. SLEEP

You sleep better on an empty stomach. Have your last meal 3 hours before you go to bed. Also a short walk before bedtime helps to settle your stomach and you sleep better. Sleep and immunity are linked.

Mammals that sleep more produce greater levels of disease fighting white blood cells – but not more red blood cells.

The Max Planck Institute for Evolutionary Anthropology has shown that species that sleep more have a greater resistance against pathogens (Obs 11/10/09).

13. HEADACHES

If you get a persistent headache, drink lots of water, it will help!

14. VITAMIN C

Because of the dramatic changes in our diet over the last 1000 years, everyone is short of Vitamin C. We all suffer from "HYPOASCORBEMIA" a lack of Vitamin C in our diet.

When we were hunter gatherers up till 10,000 years ago, 80% of our diet was raw green "stuff". We get only a tiny fraction of that in our modern diet and we all suffer its lack.

To begin with take a gram of buffered Vitamin C with every meal. This can be any proprietary brand as long as it contains 1000mg of Vitamin C plus bioflavonoids (i.e. Rose hip powder, citrus and etc.) You will begin to look and feel better within a week and will suffer less colds and minor ailments. Later you can increase this dosage to suit yourself. I take at least 5 a day and have done for 30 years. (More on Vitamin C later.)

15. MINERALS

The soil from which our food is produced is fertilized and irrigated to produce crops year after year. Thus the mineral load that healthy soil carries is reduced year after year and not replaced.

The food produced in this way looks great but contains far less goodness in the form of the micro nutrients and minerals that we need for full good health and vitality.

To counter this I take a mineral supplement containing chelated calcium, magnesium and zinc each day. I strongly recommend that you do the same. I also take a selenium tablet and a 400 iu Vitamin E capsule.

16. PROPOLIS

Propolis tincture (in alcohol) is very good indeed to help cure mouth ulcers and mouth sores. "Dab" it on with an ear bud and gargle with a few drops in warm water before going to bed. Your ulcer and sores will soon disappear.

Propolis is what the bees use to protect their hives. It is made by them from tree balsam and plant wax. It is the best natural antiseptic in the world and if you can buy some of the actual propolis, chewing it will keep your mouth sweet and healthy.

17. VITAMINS

Our diet no longer contains the range of vitamins, minerals and enzymic complexes it once did when we were hunter gatherers. So we miss out on a high proportion of the 700 or so herbs, nuts, berries, fruit, shoots and roots we are adapted to thrive on.

I try to replace these, to some extent, by taking a multivitamin supplement made from plants grown and harvested from unpolluted soil. I use Floravital or Floradix (if you need iron). This is a liquid and very easy to assimilate. I recommend it as it's the best out of all the multivitamin preparations I've tried and doesn't use any chemicals other than what the lifeforce put into fresh healthy plants.

18. LAVENDER OIL

Lavender oil applied sparingly will dry up cold sores. Also, if you dab it on to almost any spot, sore or skin infection it helps clear them up really quickly.

Lavender oil is one of the best all round healers in natures store.

If you burn yourself, quickly cover the burn with Lavender oil – it not only helps the healing process but it stops the pain almost instantly. Also, Lavender oil is very useful on insect bites.

19. CHARCOAL

There is a form of charcoal C60 which is called Buckminster Fullerene because of the shape of its molecule, which is geodesic i.e. like a football. This is the most biocompatible substance in creation and is what you, and all other living creatures, are made of. Because it is full of cracks and fissures it has a huge surface area and this can adsorb, i.e.bind to itself, most poisons and almost 4000 known toxins. I take 4 capsules daily to keep my toxin levels down. I recommend that you do the same and increase the dose if you get an upset stomach – it helps!

Charcoal can also reduce cholesterol thus reducing the need to take statins which I have found to have dangerous side-effects (i.e. they block the body's production of vital CoQ10's).

This helps clear up your system reducing the load on your liver and kidneys, also your complexion improves! It also purifies the blood, they give charcoal to people who have overdosed on drugs as it takes the drugs out of their systems and blood stream.

20. NEG IONS

A negative ionizer on your bedside table will help you breathe clean air because it neutralizes all the positive ions which attach to dust particles and cause them to plate-out onto the nearest surface. Stand it over a piece of white paper and see the grime build up. You'll be amazed at how much dirt we breathe in at night! A negatively ionized atmosphere reduces the levels of serotonin in your blood rendering you more calm – you sleep better and breathe better.

This helps asthmatics very much and used to be sold as a cure for asthma because it works.

The white blood corpuscles pick up the negative ions in the air distributing them around the body where they assist cellular respiration. This promotes faster healing, more rapid growth and more vigour. Play the neg-ion plume onto a burn and it calms down and heals faster.

Walk in the rain and breathe deep, it's full of negative ions. So is the air at the seaside or beside waterfalls.

Reference *The Ion Effect* by Fred Soyka with Allan Edmonds. Bantam Books E.P. Dutton & Co. Inc ISBN 0-553-12866-3.

21. SHOWER

A Shower is more refreshing than a bath because by splitting the water droplets into smaller units the shower bead causes them to take up a slight negative charge. These negative charges (negative ions) act to calm and rejuvenate you because they neutralize the positive charge you pick up from your environment (friction is part of this build up).

Baths are very calming but showers are better at helping you become more vigorous. At the end of a hot shower turn it to cold for several seconds. This closes the pores and brings the warm blood to the surface of your skin HELPING YOU FEEL GREAT AND IMPROVE YOUR CIRCULATION AND THUS YOUR COMPLEXION.

22. SIESTA

A Siesta after lunch is very good for you. It lowers your blood pressure, improves the depth of your respiration and thus reduces the lactic acid level in your blood, reducing fatigue.

A siesta also improves your mental state, reducing stress and tension. Even as little as a ½ hour snooze after lunch is very beneficial and helps considerably with your digestion. With the advent of TV we all stay up later and sleep less than previous generations. This is one of the reasons for epidemics of illness. You need rest!

Enjoy a siesta and live better, you'll have much more energy for important things in your life and you'll feel better, look better and last longer!

23. TOOTHPASTE

Most toothpaste contains Sodium Laureth Sulphate, a substance used in rat poisons! Plus several other things you wouldn't knowingly put in your mouth or certainly not regularly.

The best toothpaste or at least the best tooth cleaner in the world is crushed sea salt mixed with hardwood charcoal. This really whitens your teeth whilst absorbing bad bacteria and helping to heal any sores or inflamed areas in the mouth.

I mix in some cloves ground into a powder, also some cinnamon. Both these spices are antibacterial and help keep your mouth and trachea healthy.

24. TAP WATER

Tap water is disinfected with Chlorine and "brightened" with Aluminium Sulphate. Chlorine is a poison gas and Aluminium Sulphate can turn your hair green before killing you. The quantities of these in tap water are very small yet drunk every day over the years their effect builds up and contributes to a weakening of your immune system.

It's better not to drink tap water but if you must, at least filter it through an activated carbon filter beforehand. If you haven't got a filter jug, you help clear these toxins out by placing a lump of lumpwood charcoal in your water jug overnight, but make sure that if you use barbeque charcoal, that it hasn't been treated with a petrol derivative to make it burn better. A clean lump of charcoal makes the water taste better.

25. BORAX

In those parts of the world where there is a significant amount of Boron in the soil the local people do not suffer from arthritis. Therefore, I take a minute amount of Borax with my food each day.

Borax, or its derivative Boron, is a trace element (metal) so I take the equivalent of 2 grains of rice in volume daily. Hardly measurable but very effective!

You can buy Borax cheaply on the internet and a small bag/box will last years.

26. HANGOVERS

After a heavy drinking session drink a pint of water and take 1 gram of Vitamin C plus 2 charcoal capsules.

The water helps flush out your system and stops the inevitable dehydration alcohol causes, the Vitamin C stimulates the complement cascade – a vital part of your immune system and the charcoal absorbs the nasty trace elements and fractional distillates present in drink. It won't absorb alcohol but it will remove the things that make you feel rough the following day.

27. ANGER

If you get angry or frustrated you need to "let off steam" otherwise you have to "digest" these emotions which take time.

Take a pillow somewhere where you can be alone (i.e. the bathroom) and have a good scream into it. Yell, scream or roar until you are hoarse – you'll feel a lot better. Alternatively, get an axe and chop wood (whilst visualizing the source of your anger) or set up a punch bag, put on some practice gloves and give it a good thumping! The exercise will do you good and you'll feel a lot better.

28. DIGESTION

Anise, Fennel, Dill and Caraway seeds can be chewed to aid digestion. They are calmative and they make your breath smell sweeter.

Pick one you like (or a complex of several) and carry them with you in a pillbox. If you can't find an adequate pillbox, a small cylindrical film container will do. Photo shops usually have bags of them to get rid of.

These seeds are the peak of the plants investment in its future and contain a spectrum of minerals and vitamins that we need to be healthy.

29. CRUDE BLACK MOLASSES

Crude black Molasses is got from sugar cane as a by product of sugar production. Sugar cane is a grass with very deep roots. They often go up to 16 feet into the earth and bring up a wonderful complex of minerals and trace elements which in these days of monoculture farming are missing from our diet.

I find it a bit strong to eat on bread, so I make a hot drink by mixing it with water, 1 teaspoon to a cup, and drinking it.

It gives your energy a boost and it also tops up your diet with the much needed trace elements.

The addition of mixing trace elements plus the alkaline input of crude black molasses can help considerably when you are recovering from life threatening illnesses.

Make sure you use crude black molasses – refined products are no good!

30. SLEEP POLARITY

Human beings are basically one-fathom-tall columns of salt water and salt water is a very good electrolyte - a good conductor.

We live in the Earth's electromagnetic field and fare better when our bodies are aligned to it.

Place your bed so that you sleep on a N-S axis so that you are parallel to the field lines entering and exiting the N & S poles. You will sleep better!

Google earth discovered that all herd animals on the planet tend to line up this way and whilst we're not necessarily the same as herd animals our blood has a high iron content and our system works better in line with the Earth's magnetic field.

31. AIDS AND HIV

All over Africa Aids is epidemic except for Senegal where the incidence is quite low. The earth in Senegal has quite high levels of selenium which is thought to confer some degree of immunity. We know that lack of selenium in a diet can lead to Goitre, so it probably has some vital, as yet undiscovered, role to play in the immune system. I take a selenium tablet every day as a food supplement (200ug is plenty) just to be on the safe side since its one of the minerals largely absent from processed foods.

Dr. Hulda Regehr Clark, PhD.ND. in her book *"The Cure for HIV and Aids"* has a very sound practical approach to these problems which works!

New Century Press, Chula Vista, CA ISBN 1-890035-02-5.

Ref www.newcenturypress.com

32. CHARGED WATER

Keep your water jug on a magnet with the North Pole facing upwards into the body of water.

The hydrogen bonds in water are constantly coming together and breaking apart in response to the fluctuations of the geomagnetic field. By subjecting your water to a close magnetic field you are helping to form longer chains of molecules which make the water easier for your body to assimilate. Making the water wetter! Which makes you better!

This marginally increases your natural energy levels over time.

33. BREAST CONGESTION

To relieve breast congestion, massage the outer length of your thigh in the direction of your heart. Also massage the inner and outer side of your arms from wrist to shoulder always towards your heart. Massage the front of your shoulder away from your heart and massage around and upwards from beneath your breast to your armpit/shoulder. Massage around your breasts in a circular anti-clockwise motion (it is not necessary to massage the breasts themselves). This is all about freeing up lymph which has become stagnant.

Wear garments that fit well, get plenty of exercise, use a rebounder. These are very good for lymphatic circulation, drink lots of water and use only natural i.e. herbal or crystal deodorants. Avoid anti-perspirants. They clog the pores and prevent toxins from leaving your lymph. Don't worry, you will soon begin to smell much nicer as your diet changes.

34. COMFREY

Otherwise known as "Knitbone" comfrey is the best remedy for bruising that I've ever come across. In the middle ages it was very widely used and formed a vital part of treatment after Agincourt.

Comfrey ointment will bring out a bruise in a very short time – with no side-effects. Even deep bruises respond well and quickly to its healing powers. The sticky brown ointment is better than the mild yellow one but both work well.

35. SEAWEED

Seaweed is the most nutrient rich vegetable you can eat. It's used widely in areas of the world like Okinawa where the people live very long and vigorous lives.

Dulse, Nori, Arami, Wakame, Kombu are all edible and very good for you. Add them to stews, soups, salads, to rice, to casseroles, in fact to almost any dish. Each has its own characteristic but all contain elements that you need and which fill out your diet making it healthier.

Seaweeds provide all of the 56 minerals and trace elements required for the body's physiological functions. They contain 10 to 20 times the minerals of land plants and an abundance of vitamins and other elements necessary for metabolism.

Nature's secret for a long and healthy life.

There is a comprehensive analysis of the benefits of Seaweed in longevity published in *The Nutrition Practitioner* 2006 Winter Vol 7 No. 3 pp 29-43 or Google 'seaweed + longevity'.

36. BAREFOOT

Our bodies function according to the rhythms of the earth and sky but we divorce ourselves from the earth by wearing rubber or leather insulators (i.e. shoes). If you walk barefoot in your garden or in the park or countryside you will become "earthed". Your mood will lighten, your blood pressure will reduce and you will feel more grounded, better able to deal with life's problems.

Go barefoot and the uneven ground massages the reflex points on your feet which helps the corresponding organs of your body to be more healthy.

Go barefoot and the "CHI" will flow more strongly through your body connecting you with the diurnal flow of energy between the earth and the sky. Set aside some time each day to quietly walk barefoot, you will feel surprisingly energised.

37. FILLINGS

If you have any mercury amalgam fillings in your teeth have them replaced with the latest "glass" or alternative fillings. The reason for this is that mercury is extremely toxic and mercury based fillings leak.

You could argue that the amounts involved are tiny and can't do much harm but that's not the point, even tiny amounts of poison can act as triggers for long-term ill-health, so why run the risk?

38. MEAT

Your digestion system has to work hard to digest meat. To do so it increases your body temperature and your heart rate. If you reduce your meat intake you will have more energy. Studies on Olympians have shown that those on a predominantly vegetarian diet have more energy, more stamina and longer endurance. They also smell better!

Much of our meat supply today is tampered with by the addition of hormones, antibiotics and strong chemicals (i.e. pesticides). These accumulate and in the long-term can have very damaging effects on our health. Wild game is relatively safe from contaminants, so if you want to eat meat, source it carefully.

39. COMPUTER SCREENS

If you regularly use a computer screen you should take regular breaks as they tire your eyes very quickly. Keep a piece of green cloth to hand. Looking at something green rests your eyes and helps them recover. This is an old marksman's trick and works vey well but the "bottom line" here is that computer screens are bad for your eyes and will, if used to excess, and over long periods, damage your eyesight!

My son, Tobias, was suffering with his

eyes which could not discern objects as clearly as before and this scary situation reversed when he went to work outdoors and got away from computer screens. He now has perfect eyesight again.

40. ENERGY FOOD

You can sprout mung beans and barley, indeed a whole range of seeds to produce edible shoots or sprouts. You first soak them thoroughly in pure water and then spread them out on a tray to sprout. (It helps them to sprout more vigorously if they are aligned north-south). As they develop over a day or two the sprout forms containing all of the food value that has been sleeping in the bean or seed, plus a huge jolt of pure energy contributed by the lifeforce. This sparkle of energy, commented on by Goethe, and the founder of Anthropology, Rudolph Steiner, has formed the basis for a healing practice which has cured a vast range of illnesses. For our purposes it delivers great energy via your much restored digestive system. Energy which tops up your flagging vitality. Try to eat a handful of raw shoots every day. You'll feel and look much better and save a fortune.

The Sprouting Book by Ann Wigmore
ISBN 0-89529-246-7, Avery Publishing Group Inc. Wayne, New Jersey.

41. TOOTHACHE

Keep a small bottle of clove oil in your medicine cabinet, it gives temporary relief from toothache.

If you get toothache and the dentist can't see you quickly, simply "dab" clove oil onto the offending area and the pain will go away for a while.

Don't put too much on as it can burn the surrounding area if it's used too often or in too strong a concentration. Just "dab" enough on to ease the pain so that you can function normally until you can see the dentist.

If you have toothache and can't get to a dentist quickly, you can achieve some relief by softening a piece of propolis in your mouth and then sticking it to the offending tooth.

Propolis is nature's top healer made by the bees from leaf wax and complex plant oils. It is used to plug gaps in their hives and to disinfect their brood. It sterilizes almost all bacteria and is wonderful for oral hygiene.

42. ACTIVATED FOOD

Most "fresh" fruit has been stored in a cool store to stop it fully ripening and then going off. So when you buy fresh fruit after washing it in a vinegar rich rinse, leave it a few days to warm up and begin to ripen. A. It tastes better when it's ripe and B. This has allowed all the digestive enzymes it contains to become active. These enzymes contribute to your body's ability to digest the fruit and help to top up your energy levels. You can tell when fruit is truly ripe by the way it smells. This ancient function of the frontal cortex of the brain is one of our most developed ancient survival skills.

43. MELATONIN

Take off your sunglasses for an hour a day when it's sunny. Your eyes need sunlight to stimulate the production of melatonin. This is the hormone that regulates many of the functions of your body, the most vital of which is your biological clock – your sleep cycle.

Just as rising levels of UV trigger plant growth in the spring, so rising levels of sunlight with all its component radiations trigger your body's responses. Sunglasses can block out much of this effect and so you will benefit from taking them off and getting a good dose of full spectrum sunlight when it's available (but please don't look directly at the sun). Get your daily dose before 11am and after 4pm, at these times its rays are filtered through more of the atmosphere and won't hurt you.

Reference The Melatonin Miracle by Dr Walter Pierpaoli 1995.

Also an excellent book:- *The Super Hormone promise. Nature's antidote to ageing* by William Regelson MD and Carol Colman – Pocket Books ISBN 0-671-01003-4.

44. SUNLIGHT

Spend as much time as possible outside in the sun. Your body needs natural sunlight to manufacture Vitamin D, a hormone which fights cancer.

It is safe to sunbathe before 11am and after 4pm since the sunlight has to pass through our fairly dense atmosphere before and after these times. In between these times always wear a hat and on hot days use a natural sunblock like olive oil if you are going to sunbathe.

Flaxseed oil and better yet Hemp oil are very good sunblocks. Hemp seed oil particularly has been shown, in an important Canadian study, to protect skin from broad spectrum UV radiation.

45. COLD FEET

If your feet are cold place them in cold water and they will warm up quickly. Sounds crazy but it works!

This is especially effective in springs or "live" water sources.

46. STEAMED VEGETABLES

Instead of boiling your vegetables, place them in a broad flat pan, put in no more than 1/8th of an inch of water and put on the lid. Bring this to the boil so that the vegetables are lightly steamed rather than being immersed in boiling water.

By this process you can, with practice, eat your vegetables when they're slightly crunchy (al dente). Also, this process keeps in them all the goodness which, if you boil them, goes into the water which gets thrown away!

The whole point of fresh vegetables is to benefit from the vitamins and minerals they contain at the peak of enzyme rich freshness.

47. FAT

Trim the excess fat off meat before you cook and eat it. Mammals are designed to store not only spare energy in fat but also it is used to store anything else in their food which cannot easily be processed or evacuated. In this way growth hormones fed to livestock end up in their fat layer, as do a range of antibiotics etc. You do not want to take on this toxic overload, so avoid excess animal fats.

48. MOBILE PHONES

Mobile phones use microwave frequencies to function. These cause hot spots to occur in your brain which give rise to mental "fogging". Use them sparingly and swap ears regularly to cut down exposure time.

Long-term exposure to microwave radiation is very dangerous and can cause sterility, as well as brain damage. Use your mobile wisely i.e. as little as possible. It's one addiction that can shorten your life significantly.

Ref. *Electromagnetic Man Health and Hazard in the Electrical Environment* by Cyril W. Smith and Simon Best ISBN 0-460-860-445 Published by Dent.

49. TRAPPED WIND

Carbo Veg is a homoeopathic remedy for trapped wind. It really works very well and can reduce the pain caused by trapped wind in minutes.

A build up of gas in the intestines can put pressure on your heart, which is something to be avoided.

Carbo Veg at a potency of 10 or as high as 30 will help you reduce wind pain (as will charcoal).

Trapped wind can contribute to heart problems when it puts excess pressure on the heart. Carbo Veg helps reduce this risk – it works!

Weleda do a good line in this and other homoeopathic remedies (which work!)

50. HUNGRY DAYS

Have a hungry day once a week when you eat little.

This rests your digestion giving it

time to catch up with all the processing it has to do. This also helps boost your immune system whose function is tied in to your digestive system. Also, you will sleep better on an empty stomach. <u>Small</u> snacks a couple of times a day, especially ripe fruit, will help keep hunger pangs at bay and you soon get used to this practice. You also feel a lot better for it (and save money).

51. TRANSFORMERS

If your bed head is near an electrical transformer, move as far away as possible. Transformers have been shown to have a link to high levels of leukaemia and in any event are worth avoiding.

Also, it is unwise to have electrical appliances switched on and plugged in close to your head at night. They need to be at least arms length away.

Electrical cables and wires have a magnetic field around them. This magnetic field attracts particles of dust, some of which plate out onto the cable or its surrounds which is why cables get dirty in time. Some of that dust is radioactive because it attracts radon gas from the air. You don't want it in your LUNGS, so keep away from electrical appliances when you are sleeping.

52. POWER LINES

If you live under or close to overhead electrical power transmission lines – MOVE!

Their signal strength ranges across a broad band of frequencies which can disrupt the body's intercellular communication causing illness, especially to sensitive people. This is very difficult and expensive to shield against, also it is insidious, why run the risk? (See Fishponds study). Ref *Electromagnetic Man* (see 48).

53. RED WINE

A glass of red wine is good for your heart, 2 are enough and 3 too many!

We have been designed by evolution to consume fermented fruit and the trace elements it carries. Up until a century ago everyone drank ale or a small beer in preference to water since the alcohol killed unwanted infection bacteria. When the temperance movement persuaded people to give up this practice a lot of malnutrition was the result. This was because abstinence removed all the vital trace elements and minerals in ale and beer from people's diets and they suffered as a result.

French studies confirm that regular red wine drinkers suffer from less heart disease than their non-drinking contemporaries. Champagne and some other sparkling wines share the health benefits of red wine.

Dr. Jeremy Spencer of Reading University, working with scientists in France, has confirmed that it is the polyphenols in red wine which help ward off heart and circulation problems by slowing down the removal of nitric oxide from the blood. Elevated levels of nitric oxide cause blood vessels to dilate lowering blood pressure and reducing the risk of strokes and heart problems.

Red wine and champagne contain polyphenols, white wine does not!

54. PANIC ATTACKS

Put 2 drops of lavender oil on your handkerchief and slowly inhale the fumes. Breathe deeply and slowly until the attack dies down.

Hum a simple catchy tune as you exhale – the mind can only really concentrate on one thing at a time, so this activity displaces the worry. I find the Beetles tune, "The Fool on the Hill" works for me but any slowish catchy tune will do.

I think it was Buzz Aldrin, but anyway one of the first astronauts used this technique (i.e. singing a simple repetitive song) to good effect during earth re-entry from space.

55. ENEMAS

Our diet and lifestyle has changed radically during the last fifty years and we no longer get the kind of exercise nor the roughage in our diet that used to keep us regular.

Also, our diet has become much richer, much sweeter, and much more salty than used to be the case. It also contains many preservatives, colourings and additives which were not there before.

Many of these pass through our systems to lodge in the lower intestine where, if not regularly evacuated, they can give rise to a host of ailments, also bad breath and poor skin condition as your body tries to expel them by other routes. It is very health-giving to have a good flush out with an enema once every so often. You will feel much lighter and better for it and your skin will clear up. You can have this done professionally at a number of Health Clinics if you are uncertain about doing it yourself.

56. MUSHROOMS

Mushrooms and fungi form the largest living structures on our planet often extending miles under the surface. Their main role is the breakdown of decaying animals and vegetation but they also collect and concentrate heavy metals in the process.

They can become dangerous to eat if there has been steady levels of radioactive fallout in an area and are best avoided if the prevailing wind blows from the direction of a nuclear facility. Better safe than sorry.

Those collected around Chernobyl are still toxic which is why the locals are prevented from gathering them – an age old pastime in those areas.

57. CACAO

Cacao is a wonderful energy rich food and eating this dark chocolate which is quite bitter is very good for you. The other soft sweet chocolate is really just a medium to get you further "hooked" on sugar and is not good for you at all in the long-term.

High levels of sugary foods admittedly give you a quick energy boost but you come down equally quickly shortly afterwards. Cacao is a very sophisticated food which delivers sustained energy over a longer period weight for weight than its lighter, cheaper relative.

Cocoa beans are high in polyphenols which lower blood pressure. So a drink of cocoa at bedtime is very good for you.

58. INSOMNIA

A lettuce sandwich last thing at night helps you get off to sleep. It can also help you get back to sleep if you wake up in the middle of the night. So use lettuce sandwiches as your midnight snacks.

Lettuce contains natural soporifics which relax you and help you sleep <u>naturally</u>.

59. ALUMINIUM

Avoid cooking in aluminium pots and pans. Aluminium can accumulate in the brain and could become a causative factor in Alzheimers.

60. COLLOIDAL SILVER

Silver has antibacterial properties. Soldiers used to swallow silver coins to help wounds heal.

Settlers crossing America used to put silver coins in milk to make it last longer. Aristocrats were said to have been "born with a silver spoon in their mouths", a reference to the food that they ate with silver utensils to cut down infections.

Silver is used very widely in water filters to cut down bacterial build up. Today silver is available as a colloid i.e. a suspension of very fine particles created by electrolysis. Colloidal silver has amazing healing properties both as a wound dressing and taken internally. It helps the immune system to overcome illness even to the extent of helping people with HIV to live more healthy lives.

Colloidal silver is an excellent mouthwash and taken regularly (i.e. twice a week) does wonders for your skin.

Please read *Colloidal Silver* by Dr Keith F. Courtenay ISBN 1-876494-10-7 Oracle Press PO Box 121 Montville Queensland 4560 Australia.

61. YOUR BOTTOM

The Gluteus Maximus is the main storage area for fat in your body and since we nowadays follow a fairly sedentary lifestyle it soon gets fat!

To reverse this process is simple:- Sit on the floor on a fairly rough rug or carpet, draw your knees up to your chest and, using your arms to support your balance, shuffle up and down the room. Do this regularly each day and the fat will melt away!

By shuffling your weight along on an area which gets very little pressure massage from exercise, you are pumping the stagnant lymph around your body, breaking down fat cells and increasing the circulation in this muscle.

The fat falls away if you do this every day.

Five to ten minutes is plenty, regularity is the secret – a little and often for the best results.

62. YOUR BACK

Back pain and bad posture are epidemic in our TV-watching, computer-driven society, yet a healthy spine is essential to full good health. Buy a rubber rugby ball, sit on the floor, place the ball behind your buttocks and lay back over it. Wait a few moments whilst your pelvis adjusts to a new posture and then roll up and down your spine on the ball. You can use your arms and legs to propel you and try to do this slowly so as to give all the spinal muscles a really good stretch – workout. This is really good for your posture and for your general health, also it promotes suppleness.

A supple healthy spine is a very youthful attribute. Reference:- *Backball* by Keith Foster. Sagax Publishing. ISBN 0-95324072X.

63. BITTER SEEDS

In the Himalayas the Hunza tribes people live very long active lives on a simple diet that contains high levels of Vitamin B17. They get this, in the main, from the apricot kernels that they eat and they harvest and consume large amounts of these bitter seeds.

Chew half a dozen of these each day. They are said to ward off cancer and they certainly deliver good, necessary amounts of laetrile (B17) otherwise missing from our diet.

As hunter gatherers we wasted nothing and would have used every part of a harvest. Certainly we need the trace minerals, vitamins and enzymes stored in these seeds – also the lifeforce.

64. GARLIC

During the 2nd World War the Russians had very little in the way of antibiotics so they used garlic.

Garlic is one of the strongest antibacterial and antifungal agents in nature's pharmacy and it has the unique advantage of working on a number of levels so that the bugs can't mutate to overcome it. Garlic in your food is a must, but if you can't manage the smell, then use garlic tablets, pearls or capsules, which have no smell.

As a method of keeping internal parasites in check, garlic is very useful. It also helps to rejuvenate your blood.

See:- *Garlic Natures Original Remedy* by John Blackwood and Stephen Fulder. ISBN 0-7137-1569-3 Lavalin Books, Link House, West Street, Poole, Dorset BH15 1LL.

65. STATIC

If you generate or pick up a lot of static electricity or if you feel exhausted and edgy when you have been a long time in a dry environment with lots of computer screens around, you may need to degauss.

Get your hair dryer, switch it on, then run the back of it over your body. This reduces your "charge" and you'll feel better.

Otherwise walk barefoot in your garden to earth yourself.

Remember all our bodily processes are electro-chemical, so in many ways we resemble large accumulators and sometimes need to discharge.

66. SUBTERRANEAN
   HOMESICK BLUES

If your house/bed is situated over a subterranean stream or energy line – move! Underground streams often give off a very high frequency signal which you can't hear but your cells can. These ultra-sonic sounds interfere with cellular communication and have been shown to increase the incidence of cancer in specific properties.

Dogs and all other animals will not sleep on these energy hot spots but cats will!

If you sleep on one such energy line you will have a much higher likelihood of becoming ill. Why risk it?

Contact The British Society of Dowsers for expert advice. They can be reached on B.S.D. 2 St Annes Road, Malvern Worcester WR14 4RG. 01684 576969.

They publish a really good magazine and have a health special interest group who will be pleased to advise on Geopathic stress.

67. REFLEX POINTS

Your feet have a complex of reflex points which correspond to the organs of your body. Through these run energy lines of CHI which modulate the counterflow of the life-forces through you.

By gently massaging these points with a wooden foot roller you can relax better and become more healthy. When you are sitting at your desk, reading in a chair or watching TV roll your feet. Pay particular attention to painful or sensitive areas as they represent organs like, for example, your stomach, where tension is interrupting the flow of CHI.

A good foot massage is very health giving for the whole mind-body-spirit complex.

68. ASTHMA

Konstantin Paulovich Buteyko (1923-2003) was a medical trainee in charge of a Moscow hospital ward when one night in 1956, he first made the connection between hyperventilation and headache. He later went on to discover the relationship between what he called hidden hyperventilation and asthma which boils down to a matter of the ratio of carbon dioxide to oxygen in the blood, which relies on the gas exchange in the lungs. His theory is that modern life acts as a stress on the human body causing a rise in the automatic breathing pattern and a drop in good health. He developed a series of techniques based on special principles of breathing, diet and exercise. This Buteyko method has had great success in controlling asthma, reversing symptoms and removing the need for medication. See article *Asthma: Ignorance or Design?* By Jennifer Stark. Nexus Magazine Vol 13 Number 1. December 2005 – January 2006 or go to http://www.nexusmagazine.com

69. HEMP OIL

Forget fish oils! Hemp oil is nature's most balanced oil for human nutrition with an approximate 3:1 ratio of linolenic acid, an omega-6, to alpha-linolenic acid, an omega 3. This oil can provide all our requirements for life due to its balanced 80 per cent EFA content. Essential fatty acids are necessary for good health and are responsible for the lustre in our skin, hair and eyes and even the clarity in our thought processes as they transfer oxygen to every cell in the body. They also lubricate and clear the arteries, strengthen immunity and help prevent viral and other threats to the immune system. The body can't make them so they must be obtained from food sources. Hemp oil is unsurpassed as a highly nutritious food. See Article:- *Hemp, the Worlds Miracle Crop* by Susanna Wilkinson. Nexus Magazine Vol 16 No. 2 February to March 2009 or go to

www.puredelighthemp.com.au

You need to incorporate this oil into

your diet to look younger – your cells need the oxygen and your body the nutrients.

70. REBOUNDER

According to N.A.S.A. "Rebound exercise is the most effective exercise yet devised by man". Dr Alexander Leaf MD in his book "Youth in Old Age" points out that 10 minutes on a rebounder will give you the same benefits as a 30 minute jog but without the skeletal shock.

Rebounding is easy and agreeable, it takes less time than most other exercises and delivers a much wider range of benefits. Because it deals with gravity, acceleration and deceleration, it stimulates a whole range of bodily functions rendering them more efficient. Beginning with as little as a minute a day rebounding exercises your vitality, strengthens your pelvic floor, burns off excess fat, improves your muscle tone, lowers your cholesterol levels, improves your circulation, improves your balance and coordination and helps slow down the ageing process. Get the book, *"Rebounding for Health"* by Margaret Hawkins published by Jardine Prentis

(UK) Ltd Burnhayes House, Silverton, Exeter Devon EX5 4BU ISBN 09520780-15. They also supply rebounders.

71. IRON FILINGS

It is better to avoid using iron or steel eating utensils since minute particles of these ferrous metals scrape off and get into your food. Lodging in your digestive tract these can cause problems as they build up throughout your life and are best avoided.

Use Bronze, or better yet, silver utensils. Bronze is soft and whilst it will hold a good edge it doesn't rust! Silver is the best as it has antibacterial properties.

72. YOGA

Different emotions cramp up different muscle groups and reduce the healthy circulation of oxygen rich blood and CHI.

This can and does lead to illness in the areas in question if not addressed.

Much of our casual language alludes to this i.e. "You are a pain in the neck", "You give me a pain" etc.

The best way to deal with these problems is to take up Yoga. In its modern form it derives from a much more ancient wisdom where there is an asana for every illness.

73. BATTER

Avoid eating fish batter as it is fried in highly unsaturated oils such as rapeseed which is cheap. Most of the cooking oils used in fast food and on sale in supermarkets are processed at high temperatures which denatures their essential fatty acids to the point where they become trans fats – basically toxins with which your body has to cope.

Ideally, food oils should always be cold pressed and kept away from heat, air and light. You would be wise to avoid cooking with oil which is presented in a clear plastic or glass bottle and which has been refined, bleached and deodorised – the same goes for margarine.

Dr Udo Erasmus in his book "*Fats that Heal, Fats that Kill*" deals extensively with a table of oils from most to least beneficial. Alive Books Canada 1993 or see his website www.udoerasmus.com or go to Nexus Volume 16 No. 2 February – March 2009 Article by Susannah Wilkinson entitled "*Hemp, the World's Miracle Crop*".

74. HEART DISEASE

The true nature of heart disease was identified in the early 1950's by a Canadian team led by G.C. Willis MD. His finding was confirmed in the late 1980's by Nobel Prize Winner Linus Pauling PhD and further confirmed by Dr Kale Kenton's team in the UK using a test group of 200 men over a three year period (1997-2000.) Heart disease is a misnomer. It is characterised by scab-like build-ups that slowly grow on the walls of blood vessels and is a low grade form of scurvy.

The underlying disease process reduces the supply of blood to the heart and other organs, resulting in angina ("heart cramp"), heart attack and stroke. The correct terminology for this disease process is "chronic scurvy", a sub-clinical form of the classic Vitamin C deficiency disease. The safe and effective answer to the most common form of heart disease – plaques forming over weak arteries – is 600ug to 1800ug of Vitamin C daily to strengthen the arteries. For a complete overview of this subject go to Nexus Vol 13 Number 1 December 2005 – Jan 2006 and read the article by Dr Owen R. Fonorow *"Chronic Scurvy and Heart Disease"* or go to www.vitamincfoundation.org

75. LIVE FOOD

Our bodies are composed of cooperating hosts of bacteria organized into various organs and circulatory systems. These derive their energy in the main from the food we eat which delivers energy via a series of enzymic reactions. As we age, and particularly if we subsist largely on a diet of processed food, our reservoir of bacterial enzymes becomes depleted. This makes it harder for us to digest our food and saps our vitality. To regain a youthful enzyme bank or reservoir, your body needs "live" enzymically-charged food with a broad spectrum of minerals. Since cooking shorts-out or destroys much of the enzymes in food it is essential to add to your diet such raw foods as you can, raw foods that have been grown either wild or in a healthy and unpolluted environment. Watercress, mustard cress, wild herbs, seaweed, very ripe raw fruit, (unsprayed), berries, nuts, lettuce, onions, wild mushrooms, indeed anything that's ripe, grown in undepleted healthy soil, unsprayed and naturally occurring will help you to recover your vital enzyme reserve.

76. FAT THIGHS, SHOULDERS AND OUTER ARMS

There are areas where there are no joints to apply flexion to the muscles so the flow of lymph around your body naturally "pools" here. To get this moving again so that it can do its job of washing away toxins and circulating energy, you should apply friction.

The best way I've found to do this is to place a rough towel on the floor, lie on it favouring the area to be treated (i.e.

thigh, shoulders, outer arms, buttocks etc). And rub the area up and down on the towel. You feel like a contortionist at first but with practice you soon find the best position for each application and you'll be amazed at how quickly the fat (and cellulite) disappear and your muscle tone improves. Always try to massage the lymph towards your heart since this helps your overall circulation. Do no more than 5 minutes a day on each area – a little and often is the key!

77. DEPRESSION

If you eat a diet laden with processed and high fat foods you are significantly more likely to get depressed. So if you comfort eat fattening foods you are only making things worse. According to a study by researchers from University College London (published in the British Journal of Psychiatry – The Whitehall II study) people who eat a diet high in pulses, nuts, fruits, cereals, fish and olive oil are 30% less likely to develop depression.

I find that it is very important to get outdoors when depressed as sunlight or, in any event, broad daylight helps stimulate the production of melatonin a hormone which helps lift the spirit. However, the best cure I know is to be amongst other people and to help them. We all need to be needed and to be engaged with life.

Walking on a windy day when there is no rain can help raise the levels of serotonin in the blood and this allays depression since it's a mood enhancer.

When you meet somebody you automatically scan the left side of their face first to ascertain their mood, their emotional state. This is called "left side bias" and is an automatic response that we share with dogs, man's best friend. This is how dogs react so quickly to your moods and empathise with you. This empathy helps a lot when you are feeling a bit down.

78. LOWER BACK PAIN

Often an indicator of constipation, lower back pain is epidemic in our sentient society. One of the best ways of relieving this is to hang upside down. I use a backswing which is the name of an incline table that you clamp your feet into and which enables you to then hang upside down. It sounds scary and it is at first but once you get the "hang" of it, it is very good for you. By stretching out your spine in the opposite direction it releases the pressure on your vertebrae and the intervertebral capsules which gives a wonderful feeling of ease. It takes the pressure off sore nerves and allows the muscles that have been clamping tight with pain to relax. This also drops back into your entire system all the sediments and toxins that have accumulated at the bottom of your arteries, veins and etc. This enables your liver to give your whole system a good clean up! Drink a litre of water after backswinging as your liver needs flushing through!

79. WROTH AND FRUSTRATION

When someone or some group of people upset you, this can build up as anger and frustration. To release this you should write them a letter. In this letter you should go into elaborate detail about how they have upset you, leaving nothing out. Really, let yourself go and tell them just what you think of them and what you'd like to do to them etc. Then carefully seal the envelope and put it in a safe place where no-one else can find it. The following day, or after the passage of a couple of days, take the letter out of the envelope and destroy it completely. Burning is best. I know it sounds crazy but believe me you will feel a lot better and, funnily enough, they will get the message. Everything we say, do, think or write is impressed on the ether and becomes part of our/their reality.

80. GOOD VIBRATIONS

The human body is composed of a host of different resonant structures which, taken together, form 7 discrete Chabras or energy centres. These are:-

Energy Centre	Keynote	Cycles/Sec	Colour
Base of spine	C	261.2	Red
Spleen	D	292.1	Orange
Solar Plexus	E	329.1	Yellow
Heart	F	349.2	Green
Throat	G	392.0	Blue
Forehead (pineal)	A	440.0	Indigo
Crown	B	493.0	Violet

This structure enables us to respond to sound/music in different areas of our body and using this knowledge you can both heal yourself and improve your moods. Sound each of these notes on a piano and then sing the same note at the same time as playing the note and after a little while you will notice that your senses are heightened or lowered in accordance with the musical note.

This then can be developed into a mood-altering, health-giving complex which is able to be developed as you begin to experiment and begin to enjoy singing.

81. WEIRD WATER

The plastics industry uses a fixative in the manufacturing process which mimics oestrogen, the female hormone. This leaches out of plastic waste and is also discharged into our water courses. The build up of this hormone in our environment is responsible for fish, molluscs, amphibians and water fowl, all producing more female characteristics, also non-viable offspring unable to breed.

This situation is escalated by "the pill" which passes through our population and enters the water system unchanged and still active. The build up of these female hormones in the environment may be responsible for what appear to be increased levels of homosexuality in the population and may also be partially responsible for the decline in birth rate we are experiencing in the west. Certainly, this is another good reason for drinking only pure spring water that is shown to be free of oestrogen if you are trying for a baby, also an excellent reason to drink only water filtered through activated charcoal.

82. HIGH ENERGY FUEL

Ubiquinone Q10 or Coenzyme Q10 is a naturally occurring substance present in all cell mitochondria which is a vital part of the chain reaction by which the body produces ATP i.e. energy. It helps prevent the natural cholesterol produced in the liver from becoming rancid and is a powerful antioxidant. When we eat a high fat, high sugar, western diet the natural production of coenzyme Q10 in our bodies can't keep up and begins to fall off. This is one of the causes of lack of energy and premature ageing. Statin drugs used widely to try to control cholesterol actually blocks the body's production of its own CoQ10. This blockage of CoQ10 synthesis causes fatigue, muscle pain and skeletal acropathy, a grave deterioration of muscle. Drug ads in Canada must carry the CoQ10 statin depletion warning. See www.vitamincfoundation.org/statin.htm or read the English translation of *Q10 – Body Fuel* by Drs Flytlie and Madsen 1994 ISBN 87-7776-056-5.

Japanese research has shown that the body can absorb CoQ10 much better when it's taken in soft capsule form Bio-Quinone. Its production in the body is also enhanced by the presence of selenium, zinc, manganese, copper, and vitamins A, C, E, beta carotene and B12. The best way to supplement CoQ10 is to eat lots of fresh fruit and vegetables and cut out fat, sugar and processed foods.

83. SUPER FOOD

Wheat seeds can be sprouted in a tray with a little water, just enough to dampen them. After a few days they sprout green shoots which can be snipped off at the base and eaten. These are one of nature's richest stores of energy and have been known to restore hair colour, skin tone and vigour. You can put these through a juicer so as to make them easier and quicker to take. The result is a thick green liquid which tastes very strong and is best drunk when holding your nose or diluted with juice. The results of this super food are well worth all the trouble it takes to get it. Wheatgrass delivers huge amounts of energy and boosts your immune system accordingly.

You can buy un-radiated wheat seeds from any good health food store and juicers are widely sold on the internet.

Wheatgrass, as with all sprouting seeds, holds the very spark of life in its structure and this gives your whole system a terrific boost.

84. STRESS

People will endure appalling hardships to achieve their goals, something they believe in, and yet if asked to endure similar suffering, will, under all other circumstances, grizzle and grumble about how stressed and unhappy they are etc. Stress therefore is largely a response to things externally imposed which we do not like. The best way to handle this is to get into action to remove or re-evaluate the cause.

Meantime, it's important to let off steam so get a punch bag and a baseball bat. Give it a good beating. This helps to release stress and put things in a better perspective so that you can move on.

The herb St Johns Wort is an excellent harmless calmative used since the dawn of time to drive off "evil spirits" i.e. bad humours!

The hormone oxytocin is released when you pat/stroke your dog. This reduces stress and makes you less susceptible to heart attacks. Therefore you live longer.

85. CALM

Half an hour's quiet prayer or meditation in the morning sets you up for the day and is worth more than any medicine. Often these days we are too much involved in life's turbulence to really enjoy its passage. Life is too much with us.

You cannot live successfully if you try to please others all the time or if you live to someone else's priorities. Without being selfish or harming others, you should decide on your own priorities and live a good life accordingly. Meditation or prayer helps clear the mind and establish a slower deeper rhythm to your life.

86. EYESIGHT

"Atheromas" or "soft atherosclerotic plaques" are the name given to the build up of abnormal formations in arteries. Atheromas in the microscopic arteries in the retina have been clearly visible to eye doctors for years and Dr Sidney Bush, D.Opt, in the Hull Contact Lens and Eye Clinic, discovered in 1999 that these atheromas can be reversed in patients instructed to take from 3 to 10 grams of buffered Vitamin C daily. Dr Bush has invented a new diagnostic technique called Cardio Retinometry[R] which he believes will revolutionise cardiology see web page:-

www.vitamincfoundation.org/bush/more.html

Quite apart from Vitamin C being able to improve eyesight, it can now be shown to cure the chronic scurvy which causes heart disease.

87. IRON APPLES

If you run out of Vitamin C when travelling or if it becomes difficult to obtain, you can use an old Ukrainian method to keep up your daily intake.

Push several iron nails into an apple, then wait until they rust, pull them out, and eat the apple. That way you get a good dose of Vitamin C, plus some iron, plus some "live" food.

I know this sounds odd but it works very well and can't harm you. The ancient Greeks used to steep their swords in water because they rusted and got a better edge in the process. Then they drank the water to ward off anaemia.

88. STIMULANTS

A slice of lemon in a cup of hot water is a great way to start the day. It cleans your palate and stimulates your taste buds and appetite.

By the time you're ready for breakfast

thoughts turn to drinks like tea and coffee, both of which contain caffeine, a strong stimulant. These are a great way to get you into gear to face the day and have a range of unseen benefits. Tea, for example, is a bactericide and helps keep your stomach healthy. It is wise to stop drinking tea and particularly coffee after 4pm. The reason for this is that your body needs time to calm down off the coffee (stimulant) high. By the time you are ready for bed you will have relaxed and will sleep better. This applies particularly to people over 50 but is a general guide for everyone.

89. MEMORY

You can physically remember everything that ever happened to you, it's retrieving your memories that is the problem. As your system cleans itself up by following this course, more enriched oxygen will permeate the blood-brain barrier and your thoughts and memories will become clearer.

To take advantage of this process you should begin to exercise your mind more. The principle of "use it or lose it" comes into play here. Learn a language, learn to play a musical instrument, take up chess, play poker, write your life story etc. In other words, take up some activity that helps with retrieval and that helps organise the vast mass of useful information you have accumulated. You are a very interesting person but nobody will know unless you tell them.

90. PROSTATE

Walnuts are a very good remedy for prostate problems because they contain complexes of orthomolecular substances (i.e. bitters) which remove parasites from the blood, lower sugar levels and combat inflammation of the urinary tract.

The similarity in shape and size between a walnut and the prostate gland first started our ancestors on using this remedy. There was then a whole branch of medicine which relied for its currency on similarity. However, this one actually works and a daily crunch of walnuts will help keep your prostate healthy. (Rebounding and walking also help considerably).

Men who walk for an hour a day are two-thirds less likely to get prostate cancer. So your two best doctors are your right and left legs!

91. THRUSH

Cranberry juice is very good at clearing up thrush infections. It can be taken orally or used in a douche to help quickly rid your body of this troublesome fungus. If you incorporate it into your diet you will never have to worry about this again, it will help you to stay thrush free.

92. SHOCK

Arnica is an excellent remedy for shock and it can also help you to recover from fatigue, particularly fatigue caused by sexual excess.

We all drive our bodies too hard nowadays so it's a good idea to keep some arnica handy to help flagging spirits recover.

Shock is a transient emotion which can best be handled by turning to familiar routines to dissipate its force. Otherwise you can talk its edge off amongst your friends.

93. CANCER

The New York Times reported in the Observer Sunday November 15th 2009, ran an article about a paper in The Journal of the American Medical Association wherein Dr Barnett Kramer, Associate Director of disease prevention at the National Institutes of Health, commented on the latest findings on cancer screening. Dr Kramer said that the latest research shows that cancer is a dynamic process requiring more than just cell mutation and needing the cooperation of the surrounding cells and even the cooperation of the whole person to develop. That is to say that the latest research shows that it is the immune system or hormone levels that can squelch or fuel a tumour. Cancer is no longer to be regarded as a linear process because it can often go into remission when a person's basic health changes for the better.

This "take" on cancer is echoed in books by Hulda Regehr Clark PhD ND...

The Cure for all Cancers, by Dr Frederick B. Levenson – *The Causes and Prevention of Cancer* ISBN 0-283-99247-6 by Dercy Weston. *Cancer: Cause and Cure* ISBN 0-9758137-0-6 and by Dr T. Simoncini (oncologist) whose book "**Cancer is a Fungus**" ISBN 88-87241-08-2 is a "must read". There are also dozens of other books by a range of specialists and some amateurs dealing with various alternatives to the present treatments for cancer when viewed from the linear perspective all of which embody one common denominator - tumours cannot grow in an alkaline environment!

94. FIZZY DRINKS

The amount of sugar in most fizzy drinks is staggering. Up to 17 teaspoons full of sugar per can. They increase obesity and rot your teeth but that's not all by a long shot. Fizzy drinks contain "empty calories", in other words when you drink them you don't feel any fuller, your appetite isn't satisfied. Yet your body still has to deal with the huge sugar rush that these drinks carry. This depletes your bile production, puts a strain on your liver and makes your system more acidic. A dangerous condition as we shall see!

95. OSTEOPOROSIS

High dose Vitamin K reduces calcium in soft tissues and is considered a standard treatment for Osteoporosis in Japan.

The vitamin acts as a hormone and helps remove calcium from soft tissues into bone. See www.lef.org/magazine/mag2010/abstracts/sep2010_Vitamin-D-K-Healing-cream-Food-sensitivities_01.htm?source=search&key=osteoporosis%20in%20Japan

96. HIGH BLOOD PRESSURE/ HYPERTENSION

Normally blood pressure elevates during times of stress (the fight or flight reaction) for short periods. This increase ensures that glucose and other nutrients enter cells in order to aid response to the stress. It is normal for the pressure to normalise after the stress event passes. Any small narrowing of the arteries has an exponential effect on hypertension and, according to discussions in the British Medical Journal, ophthalmologists have noticed that the plaques form in microscopic retinal arteries before the onset of elevated blood pressure.

Linus Pauling's high Vitamin C/lysine protocol has proved extremely effective in combating high blood pressure (and details of this are available on www. paulingtherapy.com). Vitamin B6 is also more effective than most prescription drugs for hypertension according to Health journalist Bill Sardi.

97. ELECTRICAL AND ELECTROMAGNETIC FIELDS AND MICROWAVES

In volume 42 No. 303 April 2009 of the magazine Dowsing Today, Mr Richard Creightmore writes a very informed and compelling article on Geopathic Stress. Based on published research by Professor OM Ghandi he details the effects of microwave, electrical and electromagnetic field exposure on human beings.

In 1990 the US Environmental Protection Agency stated: "In conclusion, after an examination of the available data over the past 15 years, there is evidence of a positive association of exposure to magnetic fields with certain site specific cancer, namely leukaemia, cancer of the central nervous system and to a lesser extent lymphomas."

You might like to read the aforementioned article which is available from the BSD. 2 St Ann's Road, Malvern, Worcs. WR14 4RG 01 684 576 969. Website http://britishdowsers.org

98. G. M. FRANKENSTEIN FOOD

In May 2009, The American Academy of Environmental Medicine called for a moratorium on GM foods stating: "Several animal studies indicate serious health risks associated with GM food consumption including infertility, immune dysregulation, <u>accelerated ageing,</u> dysregulation of genes associated with cholesterol synthesis, insulin regulation, cell signalling and protein formation, and changes in the liver, kidney, spleen and gastrointestinal system."

According to a study published by the Union of Concerned Scientists this year, GM seeds do not produce higher yields than conventional seeds. They also pose serious ecological risks, especially from genetic contamination from pollen. (Source Isabella Kenfield, Counterpunch 14 August 2009).

99. GRIEF

Beyond sadness, grief is like a dagger to the heart, almost insupportable. Time is the only healer but you can help yourself in a variety of ways.

A strong religious belief helps to take some of the sting out of grief but if you don't have this and its associate rituals to fall back on then you might benefit from these:-

1. A Celtic "wake" for the departed where all their friends and family gather to celebrate their lives "fair takes the sting out of the thing".

2. Routine tasks preferably involving lots of other people, help to ease the burden.

3. Taking out the pain, anger and frustration on some inanimate object (i.e. a punch bag) helps in the dissipation of the energy.

4. Crying provides a natural safety valve.

5. Sex leading to emotional release is useful, so is hugging!

6. Planning for the future with friends and family helps.

Above all you should avoid taking <u>any</u> life decisions (i.e. marriage, change of career etc) for one whole year. Deep grief takes this long to heal.

Ten per cent of people who grieve become permanently depressed, and recent studies in the USA, published in the December edition of the New Scientist, show that these poor souls respond well to psychiatric techniques used to help lift depression. Worth a try "if your woe won't go!"

Grief is about sadness, but it's also about anger, disappointment and fear. Come to terms with each of these and you will feel better.

100.   FISH

Giant Gyre, which are whirlpool structures that occur in all the oceans of the world, collect debris. Most of this is plastic waste, discarded by every country in the world, which ultimately finds its way into these huge swirling oceanic garbage patches. Plastic ultimately degrades into tiny fragments present in their trillions in the oceans.

PCB's, DDT and other toxic chemicals cannot dissolve in water but the plastic absorbs them like a sponge. Fish that feed on plankton ingest the tiny plastic particles and the toxins the plastics have absorbed leach into the fish. When a predator, i.e. a larger fish or a person eats the fish that has eaten the plastic, then higher concentrations of toxins can accumulate in the body.

It may be wise to limit the amount of fish you eat and perhaps take a couple of charcoal capsules afterwards to help soak up any toxins you may have inadvertently taken in. (Source the Algalita Foundation).

101.   MULTIPLE SCLEROSIS

We naturally produce some Vitamin D in our bodies in response to sunlight – the rest of our needs which are quite high, come from our diet.

Unfortunately, most of us don't get nearly enough daylight, let alone sunlight, since we spend most of our lives indoors. Also the paucity of naturally occurring vitamins in our diet leaves us short.

Vitamin D helps prevent multiple sclerosis and may well have a role in its treatment. (Source: You Tube ref Ryan McLaughlin, Glasgow. Scottish NHS).

Supplement your diet with a tiny amount of Vitamin D to be on the safe side.

An Italian doctor, Paolo Zamboni, has developed a new theory as to how to treat MS. He postulates that MS is a chronic cerebrospinal nervous insufficiency and has pioneered a simple operation to unblock restricted blood flow out of the brain.

More than 90% of people with MS

have some sort of blockage in the veins that drain blood from the brain and Dr Zamboni believes that iron builds up in the brain blocking these crucial blood vessels. As the vessels rupture they allow iron and immune cells to cross the blood brain barrier into the cerebrospinal fluid. Once the immune cells have direct access to the brain they begin to attack the myelin sheathing of the cerebral nerves and MS develops.

Dr. Zamboni has a 73% cure rate with his operation!

102. RELIGION

Religion has all the hallmarks of an evolved behaviour, meaning that it exists because it is favoured by natural selection. Over the millennia people have become endowed with a genetic predisposition to learn the religion of their community just as they learn the language, its culture not genetics that then supplies the content of what is learned.

Religion serves as a sort of invisible government binding people together committing them to their community's needs ahead of their own self-interest. Its staple function is patching up the moral fabric of society, providing an agreed social matrix.

A strong religious belief helps to keep you healthy, for example, Christian Scientists statistically get ill less frequently than other people. Also, actuarial tables show that people tend to wait until after Christmas to die. Ergo belief affects longevity.

103.   SAD

Seasonal affective disorder is a condition brought about by too little exposure to sunlight.

In the winter when the UV content of sunlight falls plants switch off and, to a limited extent, so do we. Many people become depressed and dejected by the lack of "brightness", suicide rates go up and generally speaking there is a glum feeling around. Fortunately, it's now possible to buy lamps that give out a spectrum of light similar to a summer's day and these give relief to the stressful feelings. Full spectrum light used for short bursts in the morning and evening can cheer you up considerably. Cheap and effective! UV light stimulates the production of melatonin, a hormone which has a role both in health and mood protection. If you lack melatonin get a sun-light!

104.   DIZZY SPELLS

Dizzy spells are usually a sign that your current diet lacks some mineral or trace element. Vega testing or muscle resistance testing or dowsing will tell you which one you are missing. I cured my dizzy spells with a course of magnesium supplements available from any health food store. You only need <u>tiny</u> doses of trace elements to get your system back in balance. The trick is to find out which one(s) are missing.

105. SLEEP DEBT

Chronic sleep deprivation is a problem most people suffer from and scientists have found that sleep deprivation affects your cognitive and physiological processes. In 2008 scientists at the Karolinska in Stockholm found that it took over a week of really good sleep (8 + hours) to begin to recover from five nights of poor sleep.

But if you know that you're going to have a series of disturbed nights you can plan to recover more quickly by "banking" extra sleep a week before. Get 10 hours a night for a week, then when you go through a sleep deprived patch you will be able to recover full mental function more rapidly when things get back to normal again!

Source: Walter Reed Army Institute of

Research, Silver Spring, Maryland. Also, Karolinska Institute Stockholm.

106.   SMILE

Smile as often as you can because there is a feedback loop to your emotions.

The more you smile, the more cheerful you feel.

107.   SLEEP SPINDLE

According to Psychology Professor James Mason, too little sleep negatively affects energy, memory, learning, thinking, alertness, productivity, creativity safety, health, quality of life and <u>longevity</u>. Rapid Eye Movement sleep which occurs later, after the deep repair sleep period, is when the neo-cortex downloads information into the sub-cortex (the conscious into the sub-conscious) updating the information held there. This download takes place in high energy bursts known as the sleep spindle during REM sleep. Without this process learning cannot take place and memory is impaired.

Eve Van Cauter, University of Chicago, found the loss of even an hour results in increased levels of the hormone cortisol and decreases in the hormone prolactin, also decreases in growth hormones.

Brain wave patterns (influenced by solar, lunar geomagnetic fluctuations) indicate that repair sleep is deeper before midnight lending credibility to the old adage that an hours sleep before midnight is worth 2 hours after midnight.

108. FIZZY DRINKS AND BRITTLE BONES

Fizziness is created by adding carbon dioxide which makes drinks acidic. It was thought that this acid was neutralized in the gut but new research by Susan New, a lecturer in nutrition at the University of Surrey, shows that it can enter the bloodstream where the body tries to neutralize it with calcium – the alkaline mineral that goes into bones. Just 2 cans of drink per day can have an effect.

The acidity of the typical western diet, low on vegetables and high in fizzy drinks and meat, may already have had a significant long-term impact on bone health and the risk is greatest for children.

Research from around the world shows that a 10-11 stone person could lose an additional 15% of their bone mass over a decade from a typical western diet!

109. HRT

A number of studies have revealed that HRT can increase the risk of heart attacks, blood clots, Alzheimers disease and cancer. There are natural ways of gaining support through the menopause – nature has provided very effective ways to help with this time in a woman's life. Detoxification can relieve symptoms dramatically. Toxins from our environment such as pesticides, heavy metals and xeno–estrogens from plastics, can interfere with the body's natural ability to balance itself.

Liquid tinctures of the herb Black Cohosh which helps to balance progesterone and oestrogen. Also Agnes Cactus, useful in the regulation of the pituitary gland which balances the whole hormone system. Sage tea for the reduction of hot flushes. Colonic irrigation can help a lot with detoxification and the menopause can become a time of change and new beginnings rather than suffering.

110.   FAT WATER

Fluoride in water and toothpaste is linked to obesity due to fluoride's effect on the thyroid gland's production of hormones controlling appetite.

Dr Barry Durrant – Peatfield, a thyroid

specialist, points out that fluoride is enzyme–disruptive and affects thyroid hormones.

Thyroid hormones rely on iodine, an element in the same family as fluorine which displaces iodine in the body leading to problems with the thyroid gland. Children can be particularly affected if their mother was short of iodine during pregnancy.

The American Federal Drug Administration requires a poison warning on all fluoridated toothpastes advising children not to swallow it. In the UK the National Pure Water Association campaigns against the use of fluoride in water, toothpaste, fertilisers and air pollution. http://www.npwa.org.uk/

111. CHORAL SINGING

Singing beneficially affects the levels of cortisol (a hormone which is part of the immune "cascade") to the extent that you genuinely feel better, emotionally uplifted after a session of singing.

Choral or group singing makes you feel needed, relied upon, part of something greater than yourself. Thus it fixes you in a matrix of emotional support which gives your life purpose, strength and position.

112.   SLEEP SLIM

Artificial light extends the day and we now sleep an average 3 hours less than we did a century ago (10 then, 7 now).

Sleep deprivation lowers the levels of the hormone leptin which can trigger the consumption of carbohydrates.

Lack of sleep can also cause levels of growth hormones to plummet by 75%. These repair hormones are secreted during the deep sleep stage and they help to maintain the proportion of muscle to fat. Too little increases fat stores.

Having less than 7 hours sleep causes blood sugar to shoot up after breakfast and remains double the level throughout the morning. This triggers extra insulin, stimulating hunger and fat storage.

Lack of sleep also increases afternoon levels of cortisol, another appetite stimulating hormone.

Finally, the more time we are awake, the more time we have to eat!

A good night's sleep (i.e. 8 hours) is a crucial part of any weight loss scheme.

NOTHING TASTES AS GOOD AS SLIM FEELS.

113. FINGERS OF FATE

Testosterone in the womb promotes the development of the areas of brain often associated with spatial and mathematical skills.

Oestrogen does the same with areas of the brain associated with verbal ability.

Interestingly, scientists at Bath University have found a correlation between those hormones and the relative lengths of the index and ring fingers. If your child has a longer ring finger, he or she is likely to be good at maths. Those with shorter ring fingers are better at reading and writing.

114. SOYA

Soya is one of the most genetically modified food plants on the planet. It is also one of those most heavily "treated" with pesticides and other sinister "agro" chemicals.

Small quantities of soya will not harm you but if it forms the bulk of your diet, it will! The Food and drug administration in the USA list soya as a poisonous plant – see their website. Cut soya from your diet and you will not only be healthier but you will also reduce the pressure on countries like Brazil to cut down rain forests to grow this "blasted bean".

Soya should not be an option for human consumption but used only as a nitrogen fixing crop in repairing soil structure. Nor should it be fed to animals as it creates too many sensitivities in the gut. (See Internet for many links on Soy).

115.   SVELTE TASTE

You only get fat from what is familiar! Taste governs familiarity. By changing your diet/habits and tastes you can change your shape!

116. BLACK SMOKE

Researchers from Imperial College London have found that even small levels of air pollution cause early death. They based their findings on long-term monitoring of air quality and national data on the cause of death.

The amount of black smoke coming from vehicle exhaust has climbed significantly over the last 30 years and black smoke and sulphur dioxide are strongly linked to early death.

The risk of early death from respiratory disease rose by 19% for every 10 micrograms per cubic metre of air increase in black smoke and by 22% for every 10 parts per billion increase in sulphur dioxide during 1994-1998. Since the clean air acts have reduced industrial air pollution transport has become the big polluter.

In traffic jams switch off the air intake – avoid enclosed spaces where traffic congestion exists – and buy an air ionizer for your bedroom and living room.

117. HYPOXIA

Analysing ice core samples from ancient glaciers we know that the air breathed by our ancestors during our long evolution contained approximately 50% oxygen. 200 years ago, the air was composed of 38% oxygen and 1% carbon dioxide. The oxygen level measured by Swiss scientists in 1945-46 was 22%. They've been carefully monitoring it ever since. The most recent measure shows 19% oxygen with more than 25% carbon dioxide. In our major cities the oxygen level can be lower than 10%! Small wonder then that most of us suffer from varying degrees of toxaemia and low oxygen levels. Common causes for this condition include the intake of devitalised food, lack of exercise, breathing polluted air, chronic stress and shallow breathing. This results in insufficient metabolism causing the body to accumulate waste products faster than it can eliminate them. These show particularly on the skin.

Pathogens (disease causing viruses, bacteria, fungi etc.) proliferate in the environment created by these conditions and in turn create disease states (flu, herpes, candida etc.) These pathogens are anaerobic and cannot survive in ideal oxygen levels.

Oxygen starvation (hypoxia) at a cellular level is the underlying cause of most serious illness today and is the main component/cause of poor skin condition.

Small wonder that most of us suffer from varying degrees of toxaemia and low oxygen levels. Both our air and, consequently, our food are short of oxygen. We've chopped down most of the forests which create oxygen, denuded the seas of life so they can't trap enough CO_2 and we annually pump billions of tons of CO_2 into the atmosphere!

118. ANOXIA

The experiments in biological time assessment pioneered by Pierre Le Compte de Nouy during the First World War demonstrate the essential relationship between oxygen and healing. de Nouy analysed the rate at which wounds heal according to the age of the wounded.

He discovered that metabolic processes reflected in the rate at which the body consumes and processes oxygen in healing, slow down with age. We have subsequently discovered that this process is reversible to a degree when higher levels of pure oxygen are made available to ageing systems which suffer from anoxia (lack of adequate oxygen).

Basically metabolism is the rate at which an organism processes oxygen in food (based on relative body weight, respiration rate, food consumption and age). Youth is characterised by a faster metabolic rate which consumes more oxygen.

119. DRYING OUT

Always drink at least 1 litre of water between meals. This provides your body with the ability to flush out toxins properly, also to lubricate the vital life processes upon which your system relies.

There are many kinds of water in your body and of particular importance is the structured water in your cells. This is the carrier of all the intercellular communications and as this dries out and/or becomes murky with pollutants, then cellular communication decreases resulting in rapid ageing.

Don't let your system dry out, or you'll die out!

120. HAIR

Hair is composed primarily of the protein keratin and grows from the base follicle. Keratin is a stable protein so whatever atoms are incorporated into it as it grows remain locked in place.

Accordingly, your hair is a linear "tape recording" of your metabolism and of what you eat.

What goes into your diet goes into your hair so eat lots of fruit, drink lots of water, cut right down on meat and fish and avoid additives, preservatives and "e" numbers as much as you can.

121.   KNOCK ON WOOD!

If you've given someone a massage or helped release tension in their neck by massaging their shoulders, then the tension can go into you. The best way to dissipate this, to get rid of it, is to bang on a hardwood surface with the flat of your hands. Pass tension out this way and you will feel much better.

122.   TREE HUGGING

A tree transports thousands of gallons of water into the atmosphere every day. Its outer layer or phloem is like a giant syphon drawing water and nutrients into its upper branches.

This vast slow flow of energy can be measured and has beneficial effects on all living creatures around it. If you are feeling down or just need to be calm, hug a tree! Sounds crazy but it feels great and after a few minutes of experiencing the lifeflow you will feel better – more at one with your nature and healthier.

123.   WATERWORLD

A brilliant Welsh scientist called Morgan has established beyond all reasonable doubt that our species evolved to walk upright because we lived for millennia on the shores of a shallow African sea and foraged for food amongst its many islands. She reasons that it is only by being supported by water that we could walk upright at first and also needed to keep our mouths and noses above the surface.

Seaweed then was well within our foraging range and it's no coincidence that seaweed provides all of the 56 minerals and trace minerals required for the body's physiological function. Seaweed contains 10-20 times the minerals of land plants and an abundance of vitamins and other elements necessary for metabolism. For a full article on the benefits of Seaweed go to the Nutrition Practitioner 2006 Winter, Vol 7, No. 3 pp 29-43 or to www.nutprac.com or ring 0118 979 8686.

124. MAGNETIC THERAPY

Magnetism is made up of two rotating fields of force which corkscrew through one another. They rotate in opposite directions and each cannot exist without the other. They are the basic forces which form all matter and drive the universe, electricity being one aspect of their function. Magnetic fields are said to sweep electrons in their passing and it is this aspect of their function that gives medical benefit. The overall directional flow of electrons influenced by a magnet is from South to North from positive to negative. Energy therefore flows into the S. pole vortex and out of the N. pole vortex. This flow of energy stimulates matter (made up of protons and electrons) into a higher state of activity and therefore energises them. All living systems gain energy from the N. polarity outflow of a magnetic field and although this is slight, yet it provides a substantial contribution to many species overall energy quotient. According to the Smithsonian, sharks, for example, obtain 60% of their energy from the earth's magnetic field! Simply put, N puts energy in and S takes it out!

125.   SUNLIGHT PROTECTION

Almost 90 scientific studies over many decades have shown that Vitamin D is the cancer–protective factor generated from direct contact with sunlight, reducing cancer risk by 50%.

A definitive carefully controlled study published in 2007 on the effects of 1000 iu/day of vitamin D (with calcium) on cancer incidence showed, after a few years, that the cancer risk was 60 per cent lower than with the placebo and 77 per cent lower when corrected for participant who had already had cancer present.

Other studies have shown equally significant associations of Vitamin D with the reduction of diabetes, number of falls by the elderly, MS and other maladies.

We all need sunlight to be healthy. The

book *The Miraculous results of Extremely High Doses of Vitamin D₃* (available as an e-book), by Jeff T. Bowles explains why.

126.   OUTCOME EVIDENCE

Many traditional health care disciplines, i.e. Chinese medicine and Ayurvedic medicine, have been validated over untold generations of trial and error. They continue to be used very effectively by billions of people in many parts of the world today which is a strong testimonial to the fact that they work.

These, and other medical disciplines, such as acupuncture, herbalism and homoeopathy, have all been subject both to rigorous scientific scrutiny as these ancient cultures have evolved their own scientific establishments and peer review medical journals or as interested groups in the west have studied and recorded their results.

Thus whilst the bulk of western medicine is concerned with the use of high-tec medicine to fight infection/disease, in a sense a war against nature itself, these modalities which treat illness in the Wisdom Way have a very high incidence of success in outcome!

127. IMPOTENCE

A problem often associated with ageing impotence can flow from hormonal changes associated with poor diet (in terms of the real food value of what you eat) plus lack of exercise, low levels of zinc and other trace elements, plus failing self-confidence.

By cleaning up your system, improving your diet and rebalancing your metabolism based upon a healthy spectrum of trace elements, you will improve your sexual health.

By reducing stress, naturally, and by getting more exercise your prowess will improve. It's useful to remember that evolution has placed your testicles outside your body for the purpose of keeping them colder than the rest of your body! Wear loose and cooler clothing and you will experience an improvement. If you want to use a stimulant, the herb Horny Goat Weed is very good and unlike Viagra has no side-effects if used sensibly and on the advice of a skilled herbalist.

128. CULTURAL ILLNESS

People prefer to shirk responsibility for their own health, preferring to call on the medical profession when they become ill. However, whilst modern medicines attack disease they must also rely on the body's own defences to help the patient recover. In many ways, modern medicine is a metaphor for war against nature battling disease etc. This has led to an outgrowth of increasingly vigorous bacterial mutations as nature seeks to evolve to combat the new medicines. So we now have Pseudomonas, C. difficile, MRSA and etc. to contend with.

Our bodies are made up of a host of micro-ecosystems that inhabit our skin, our respiratory, digestive and genito-urinary systems. If we interfere with these balances by introducing antibiotics they become profoundly disturbed and take some time, if ever, to fully re-establish themselves.

The cornerstone of good health is a healthy lifestyle! This includes eating a healthy diet, getting enough sleep and exercise, avoiding stress, maintaining a healthy weight, avoiding toxic exposures, supporting detoxification and, most important of all, having a meaningful purpose in life.

129.   BAD FATS V. GOOD FATS

Denatured fats and oils that have been treated to avoid rancidity are very dangerous poisons. These trans fats lodge in our cells preventing the transportation of essential oxygen in the process of oxidation, the most important moment-to-moment living process in the body (i.e. the burning of food to produce the energy required for life).

These poisonous fats block the activity of the essential fatty acids we need in our diet and are the major cause of advanced or accelerated ageing associated with the western diet of today.

Essential fatty acids govern growth, vitality and mental state. They act like oxygen magnets or sponges that pull oxygen into the body. A high oxygen content ensures immunity to viruses, fungi and bacteria.

A balanced intake of EFA's produces smooth, velvety skin, increases stamina, speeds healing, increases vitality and brings a feeling of calmness.

Source:
www.puredelighthemp.com.au

Other source:
www.cancerfightingstrategies.com

130.   RADIATION

Phytonutrients, digestive enzymes and lifeforce properties all inhabit fresh fruit and vegetables but are destroyed by heating or irradiation.

Every living vegetable is a powerhouse of disease fighting medicine. Broccoli and celery prevent cancer, beet greens clear the liver, cilantro removes heavy metals, berries prevent heart disease, dark leafy greens help prevent over a dozen serious health conditions whilst boosting immune function and helping to prevent other infections. Black raspberries reverse oral cancer, pomegranates halt prostate cancer, green tea prevents breast cancer and so on. There are thousands of stories dealing with the disease fighting properties of foods.

Most of these healing properties are destroyed by pasteurization and irradiation.

By all means, carefully source and wash your food thoroughly but don't kill all the goodness in it. Dead food leads to dead people! www.naturalnews.com

131. THE PROBLEM

We are daily exposed to 20,000 chemical compounds which we did not evolve with! We have absolutely no idea what the long-term effects of these compounds are and even less idea of what their synergistic effect is (what effect they have when working together).

It is very important to your health and in particular to your ageing, that you either avoid or take great care to protect yourself when using any chemical. Benzine, for example, is deadly stuff and should not be allowed in contact with the skin or respiratory tract. Similarly, manufactured surfactants strip the skin of its natural protective oils encouraging premature ageing and ill-health, so you must wear rubber gloves when washing up or handling any kitchen chemical.

By stripping the protective waxes from the surface of the leaves and stems of plants, surfactants (i.e. detergents) kill them by allowing bacterial and fungal infections to penetrate their defences – same goes for humans!

132. GM FOOD

Dr. Gilles – Eric Seralini of the University of Caen has examined raw data published by Monsanto on its Genetically Modified crops. In an article reported both in the *New Scientist Magazine* and the *International Journal of Microbiology*, he states that "statistically significant signs of liver and kidney damage occurs in rats fed the maize for three months". The analysis concluded: "These substances have never before been an integral part of the human or animal diet and therefore their health consequences for those who consume them, especially over long time periods, are currently unknown."

Why run the risk?

133.   CHEMICAL COOKWARE

Perfluorooctanoic acid present in Teflon coatings on non-stick cookware becomes unstable at high temperatures. U.S. safety chiefs have linked them to cancer and manufacturers have agreed to phase them out by 2015. Now British researchers at the University of Exeter and the Peninsula Medical School have indicated a possible link to thyroid disease. The thyroid hormone system is essential for maintaining heart rate, regulating body temperature, and supporting metabolism, reproduction, digestion and mental health. Tamara Galloway, Professor in Ecotoxicology at the University of Exeter, said "Our results highlight a real need for further research into the human health effects of low level exposures to environmental chemicals that are ubiquitous in the environment and people's homes".

Why not use iron or steel cookware and avoid the risk?

134. SOCIAL NETWORKS CAN MAKE YOU FAT

Human beings have evolved to live their lives embedded in social networks. We cooperate rather than compete and statistically we are all no more than six links away from being connected to everyone else in the world.

However, networks have a hitherto unknown diversion. Using modelling techniques Drs Nicholas Christakis and James Fowler, Professors at Harvard and San Diego respectively, have shown that networks can make you fat, happy, unhappy and etc. In their book, *"Connected" "The Amazing Power of our social networks"* (Harper Press) they demonstrate that if a friend of one of your friends gets fat (i.e. someone you don't know and may never know) then you are much more likely, 20% more likely, to get fat!

Last year the Proceedings of the National Academy of Sciences published its first study of the network genetics, suggesting that about 30% of our social ties to others may be embedded in our DNA.

135.   JET LAG

Deadly organophosphates such as tricresyl phosphate (TCP) are added to aircraft engine oil to make the engines run better. The oil seals on aircraft are designed to allow a little amount of oil to pass through the seals to provide lubrication. Compressed air from the forward section of the planes engines is used to provide air for the cockpit and cabin (this is known as "bleed air"). When the air and engine oil mix a highly toxic cocktail of gases enter the lungs of aircrew and passengers (a "fume" event) causing serious long-term illness. University College London calculated in 2006 that 196,000 UK passengers are exposed to toxic gases each year, yet bleed air lines are not filtered.

For more information which may

be critical to your survival contact the Aerotoxic Association on www.Aerotoxic.org. The UK Committee on Toxicity reckons that over 600 flights a year are affected but in fact it's every flight! Jet lag is not entirely due to changing time zones but also the air supply.

High fructose corn syrup came on the market in the early 1970's and, because it's cheap and sweeter than sugar, has become the main sweetener in soft drinks, baked goods, bread, cereals, canned fruits, jams, jellies, dairy deserts and flavoured yoghurts. It now accounts for over half the refined sweeteners in the average diet. Like sugar, it has only empty calories and is highly addictive. So April 2004 Bray and others authored a paper in the American Journal of Clinical Nutrition which publicised the theory that high fructose corn syrup is more likely to cause weight gain than sugars. They cited a 2002 paper in "Diabetes" published by Taff and others which showed that a high fructose consumption lowered plasma insulin and leptin concentrations and increased triglyceride levels in women. Because insulin and leptin act as key signals to the brain in the regulation of food intake and body weight, dietary fructose may contribute to increased energy intake and weight gain. Fructose in fruit, which forms part of our natural diet, is bound to other sugars and is part of a complex that includes fibre, fatty acids, vitamins and minerals. Most of the fructose in fruit is in the form of laevulose (L-fructose) but the fructose in high fructose corn syrup is a different isomer (D-fructose). This has the reverse isomerisation and polarity of a refined fructose molecule and is therefore not recognised by the human Krebs cycle for primary conversion into blood glucose.

Therefore it cannot be used for energy utilisation, instead it's turned directly into triglycerides and body fat. Chronic high triglyceride levels translate into increased insulin resistance, inflammation and heart disease.

137.   SWEET AND DEADLY

The same goes for agave 'nectar' a newly created sweetener developed in the 1990's. It's not made from the sap of the agave or yucca plant as claimed, but from the starch and inulin of its giant pineapple shaped root bulb. High fructose corn syrup and agave nectar are both made the same way using a highly chemical process with genetically modified enzymes. Also using caustic acids, clarifiers, filtration chemicals and so forth in the conversion of the agave root starches. The saponins found in many varieties of agave plants are toxic steroid derivatives capable of disrupting red blood cells and producing diarrhoea and vomiting.

While high fructose agave syrup won't spike your blood glucose levels, it can cause mineral depletion, liver inflammation, hardening of the arteries, insulin resistance leading to diabetes, high blood pressure, cardiovascular disease and obesity.

Good health depends on wise food choices and wise food choices depend on constant vigilance.

138.   ALCOHOL AND ALLERGIES

If you struggle through the allergy season you may want to lay off alcohol for a while! Studies have found that alcohol can cause or worsen symptoms of asthma and hay fever and this is because beer, wine and liquor contain histamine, a complex chemical produced by yeast and bacteria during the fermentation process. Histamine sets off the allergy symptoms. Wine and beer also contain sulphites which are another group of compounds known to provoke asthma and other allergy-like symptoms. A study published in the journal "Clinical and Experimental Allergy in 2008" found that having more than 2 glasses of wine a day almost doubles the risk of allergy symptoms!

139.   SYMBIOSIS

In 1989 David P. Strachan published in the British Medical Journal an article dealing with the hygiene hypothesis. This postulates the theory that many modern illnesses are the result of inappropriate auto-immune responses.

The development of chlorinated drinking water, vaccines, antibiotics, and the sterile environment of early childhood have, the argument goes, as well as preventing infection, also upset the body's internal ecology. Inflammatory responses that evolved through millions of years in the certain presence of parasites and bacteria have been thrown wildly out of kilter in their absence, causing auto-immune illnesses in which the body's immune system turns on itself, and over-sensitivity to harmless antigens such as pollen, or dust, or cats, or particular food groups develops.

In the 1980s, whilst in the field in Papua New Guinea, Professor David Pritchard noted that patients infected with the necator Americanus hookworm were rarely the subject to the whole range of auto-immune illnesses. In the years since Pritchard developed a thesis to support this observation through painstaking clinical trials (which began after he infected himself with 50 hookworm). The thesis proved that the hookworm, in small numbers, seemed to be able to regulate inflammatory immune responses in their hosts. Dr. Rick Maizels PLS, at Edinburgh University, has subsequently identified the process involving the white T cells in the blood that regulate immunity, which allowed this to happen.

So it appears that a minor infestation of hookworm can actually protect us from a wide range of illnesses (probably including MS), since that is how we evolved.

There was a very good article about this in the Observer Magazine on the 25th May. It was entitled "An End to Allergies". This could be a ground-breaking development in health preservation, even if it sounds a little yucky to have to infect yourself with hookworm.

140.   END OF LIFE ANXIETY

Consciousness is eternal and ever changing. It flows through endless lives like the waves on the ocean, each similar but different.

Spirit is movement in the ether spiralling into matter for a time to electrify its identity before returning once more into the ocean of energy. Change is eternal, each affecting the other in the constant kaleidoscope of being. The illusion of individuality contorts our reason and deludes existence with loneliness and sorrow.

Loves eternal constancy is unrequited by time whose existence is only "manifest material".

Reality is oneness where we all exist.

There is no death only change!

141.   THE LIFEFORCE

Energies from the Sun, the Earth and the Cosmos set the electrons in living systems resonating.

When we eat these living structures and combine them with oxygen, we act as antenna resonating with these life creating energies. "As above so below but in a different fashion."

In growing cells there is a dipolarity between the electrically positive nucleus and the electrically negative cell membrane. This facilitates the flow of electrons which provides the energy for cell division replacement and growth.

Our bodies are in a constant re-growth process, when this process is interrupted we begin to die. In other words, when our systems get clogged-up and polluted they can't operate properly and begin to shut down. They can no longer harmonize with the life force, no longer support its energy flow!

Anything alien to the body affects this metabolic process and accelerates ageing.

SATIS

I have written this short guide to Health as a precursor to 'Harmonic Power', a philosophy of living, which incorporates ancient wisdom and modern science in such a way as to empower and enrich seekers of wisdom and truth.

Harmonic Power demonstrates how our ancestors lived lives of awesome length (and in good health). How they draw energy from the earth itself, both to construct their huge engineering projects, and to strengthen their life forces. Also, how they created a stable and just society which endured for over 30,000 years.

Transported into the modern world, Harmonic Power demonstrates a way of living in practical terms, which enables you to live a longer richer life.

As you become adept at using your Harmonic Power, you are able to avoid colds, avoid arthritis, avoid heart disease, avoid diabetes, avoid cancer avoid MS, cease to be obese (or overweight) and live a longer, fuller life. As you progress you will begin to look and feel years younger, and you will age more slowly. You don't become superhuman but rather superior human, living in Harmony with the life force.

When, in the fullness of your years you go Yonder to join your friends and relatives who have gone before, you will not be afraid but will embrace the change to a different frequency with equanimity and calmness.

Harmonic Power delivers a better life, much more energy and a clear (science based) understanding of life's continuum.

For further information please go to www.harmonicpower.co.uk

Lightning Source UK Ltd.
Milton Keynes UK
UKOW03f1000050114

224003UK00001B/1/P